Post-Polio Fatigue

A Food-First Plan for Energy, Sleep, and Daily Function

mf

Disclaimer

By reading this guide, you are accepting the terms of this disclaimer in full. If you do not agree with these terms, please do not read or use this guide.

All content within this guide is provided for informational and educational purposes only and should not be considered medical, psychological, or other professional advice. The author is not a doctor, physician, psychologist, psychotherapist, counselor, or licensed healthcare provider. Reading or using this guide does not establish any form of a patient-client or therapeutic relationship.

Always consult with a physician, licensed therapist, or other qualified health professional regarding any questions or concerns you may have about your physical or mental health. Never disregard professional advice or delay seeking it because of something you have read in this guide.

The information presented in this guide is based on general research, personal interpretation, and publicly available sources. While reasonable efforts have been made to provide accurate and current information, the author and publisher make no representations or warranties about the completeness, accuracy, reliability, or suitability of the content. The author and publisher shall not be held liable for any errors, omissions, or outcomes related to the use of this guide.

You acknowledge that you are solely responsible for how you choose to use the information in this guide and that any actions you take based on this content are undertaken at your own risk. The publisher shall not be liable for any loss, injury, or damages arising from the application of any information provided herein.

This guide does not promise or guarantee any specific result, outcome, or improvement in well-being, mental health, or nervous system regulation. Individual results may vary.

Where applicable, any tools, concepts, or names mentioned are the property of their respective owners and are used strictly for identification or illustrative purposes. Their mention does not imply endorsement. Any individuals shown in the cover or promotional images are stock photography models, and image rights have been obtained through appropriate licensing agreements.

Table of Contents

Introduction: Navigating Post-Polio Fatigue Through Everyday Choices

Living with post-polio syndrome (PPS) often means facing ongoing fatigue, disrupted sleep, and reduced energy levels—challenges that can impact independence, emotional well-being, and quality of daily life. For many individuals with a history of polio, these symptoms are more than occasional setbacks. Fatigue in PPS is persistent, can intensify over time, and often comes alongside muscle weakness, joint pain, and other complications that restrict comfort and activity levels. Trouble sleeping is also widespread, further reducing resilience and making each day more unpredictable.

If practical, tailored strategies aren't in place, post-polio fatigue can quickly become overwhelming. A lack of supportive systems can set off a cycle where exhaustion increases, the risk of injury from falls or overexertion climbs, and both patients and caregivers grow frustrated or anxious about even the simplest routines. Without clear, accessible tools, managing PPS may feel like a constant struggle—one that eats away at self-confidence and hope for improvement.

This guide is designed to shift that experience. Instead of generalized advice, it provides concrete, everyday tools rooted in food and habit changes. The goal is to help you develop a realistic, personalized plan that makes day-to-day living more manageable and less exhausting. By focusing on small but effective adjustments—whether in meal timing, hydration, snack choices, or kitchen organization—you can gradually restore a greater sense of balance and control. These strategies are drawn from the lived expertise of post-polio survivors, evidence-based nutrition guidelines, and input from leading PPS clinicians and support networks.

It's important to clarify what this guide offers and what it does not. Here, you won't find promises of a cure, recommendations for advanced or experimental medical treatments, or detailed discussions of exercise science or pharmaceuticals. The information in these chapters is meant to complement, not replace, clinical care or guidance from your trusted health team. Readers are encouraged to consult with their physicians and specialists before making any significant changes to their routine.

What you will find are actionable resources designed for your unique circumstances. Expect checklists to help track fatigue and spot patterns that might otherwise go unnoticed. There's a food-first meal-planning toolkit to simplify decisions at the fridge or pantry. Dietary rules tailored to the energy demands of PPS are included, alongside symptom management routines that help distinguish between regular tiredness and red-flag warning signs. You'll find frameworks for better sleep, hydration protocols to match your mobility and swallowing needs, and snack strategies tiered for energy stability. There are even step-by-step systems for organizing your kitchen, collaborating with caregivers, and adjusting your routine on challenging days—all engineered with accessibility and simplicity in mind.

Throughout the guide, you'll encounter practical examples, detailed charts, and user-friendly templates—every tool vetted specifically for people living with PPS and those supporting them as caregivers. Whether you are newly adjusting to post-polio fatigue or searching for ways to refine your long-standing routine, this resource aims to build your confidence. Each chapter empowers you to take sustainable steps: not by striving for perfection, but by making thoughtful choices that add up to genuine improvements in daily function and well-being.

Identifying Your Unique Fatigue Patterns (Fundamentals)

Understanding and managing fatigue is at the heart of living well with post-polio syndrome (PPS). Fatigue in PPS isn't just about being tired—it's often unpredictable, multi-layered, and unlike the ordinary tiredness most people experience. It can wax and wane through a day, sometimes coming on suddenly, triggered by activities or circumstances that may not bother others at all. Because fatigue can be so variable and influenced by multiple factors, the first step toward meaningful management is recognizing your own unique patterns. This chapter guides you through five practical tools to help you identify, track, and summarize your fatigue experience. Equipped with these strategies, you—and your support circle—can begin to make more informed, life-affirming choices each day.

Daily Fatigue Logging Checklist: Laying the Foundation

A daily fatigue logging checklist is one of the simplest and most effective starting points for gaining control over PPS fatigue. Regular tracking can help you uncover otherwise hidden connections between your activities, environment, emotions, and the timing or severity of your fatigue. By recording your observations consistently, you create a clear record you can share with healthcare professionals, caregivers, or use for your own insight.

Here's what to include on your daily fatigue logging checklist:

- ***Time***: Note the specific times when you feel waves of fatigue, including when you first notice changes and when symptoms peak.
- ***Triggers***: Identify what might have brought on the fatigue. Was it a physical activity, emotional stress, weather change, skipped meal, or anything unusual in your routine?
- ***Severity***: Use simple ratings such as mild, moderate, or severe. You might also use a 1-10 scale if you prefer more nuance.
- ***Associated Activities***: Record what you were doing immediately before and during the onset of fatigue. Daily life tasks, nutrition choices, conversations, or rest periods can all matter.

This tracking process does not require elaborate tools. Many people use a small notebook, pre-printed forms, or dedicated smartphone apps—whatever is most accessible and easiest to use throughout your day. The key is regularity. Over just a week's worth of tracking, you will likely notice repeating themes that can inform steps to adjust your activities or seek extra support .

Practical Example:

Consider Marlene, who found her fatigue often worsened after breakfast and peaked mid-afternoon. Through daily tracking, she realized that both overnight sleep disruption and skipping her mid-morning stretch contributed to these low points. This discovery allowed her and her caregiver to rearrange the timing of meals and rest to maintain steadier energy.

Weekly Symptom Pattern Chart: Visualizing Energy Highs and Lows

While daily logs provide detailed "snapshots," a weekly symptom pattern chart brings your data together to reveal broader trends. By visualizing high- and low-energy intervals across your typical routines, you can better anticipate challenging periods and plan accordingly.

Here's a straightforward process for building your weekly chart:

Draw a table or grid with days of the week along one axis and common time blocks (e.g., early morning, mid-morning, lunch, afternoon, evening) along the other.

For each block, use a color code or symbol system (such as smiley faces, checkmarks, or shaded boxes) to represent your overall energy/fatigue severity, referencing your daily logs.

Make brief notes in each box about significant fatigue triggers, successful coping strategies, or unusual events.

Review the chart at week's end, looking for repeating "low points" or "energy windows."

Table 1: Weekly Fatigue Chart

	Early Morning	Mid-Morning	Lunch	After noon	Dinner
MON					
TUE					
WED					
THU					
FRI					
SAT					
SUN					

This summary makes it easier to plan critical tasks during higher-energy periods, schedule appointments, or coordinate caregiver visits for times when you're most likely to need help. It also provides a valuable overview to share with your health team, reducing the need to remember every detail during appointments.

For visual learners or anyone who feels overwhelmed by written logs, a chart or even stickers on a large wall calendar can be especially helpful. Over several weeks, you'll notice not only the effects of specific days (such as the week after increased physical activity), but also the influences of weather, meal patterns, or stress events on your energy.

Top 5 Environmental and Emotional Fatigue Amplifiers Worksheet

Fatigue in PPS is rarely the product of a single factor. Instead, it results from a combination of physical, environmental, and emotional triggers—which can change from day to day. Identifying your top fatigue amplifiers specific to PPS can help you take active steps to minimize their effects or avoid them when possible.

Here, a worksheet approach can help distill these patterns:

- ***Environmental Triggers***: Review your weekly charts and daily logs for places or circumstances that make fatigue more likely. These often include high temperatures, poor ventilation, loud noises, poor lighting, or the physical layout of home and work spaces. For example, tasks requiring frequent standing or trips up and down stairs are common culprits.

- ***Emotional Triggers***: Fatigue can be magnified by feelings of anxiety, frustration, social isolation, or sadness. Even positive stress—such as excitement over a family event—may tip the balance.
- ***Nutrition and Hydration***: Skipping meals, inadequate fluid intake, or consuming foods low in iron and other nutrients can aggravate fatigue and hinder muscle recovery.
- ***Sleep Disruptions***: Noisy environments, pain, or anxiety can interrupt restful sleep, leading to "carryover" fatigue the next day.
- ***Overexertion***: Pushing physical limits, often in an attempt to "catch up" on tasks, can trigger delayed and prolonged fatigue.

Your worksheet might look something like this, with each row representing a category and space to list your own top examples:

Table 2: Worksheet

Environmental (e.g., excessive heat in the afternoon)	
Emotional (e.g., increased family stress on weekends)	

Nutrition (e.g., skipped lunch or low-iron meal)	
Sleep disruptions (e.g., woken by pain at night)	
Physical overexertion (e.g., standing too long while preparing meals)	

Periodically reviewing this worksheet can help you and your support team focus on changes likely to make the biggest difference in your everyday energy levels.

"Red Flag" Fatigue Signals Decision Matrix

For individuals with post-polio syndrome, some forms of fatigue signal the need for rest, while others act as "red flags" that may require clinical attention. Differentiating between these can prevent complications and support timely intervention.

Building a decision matrix helps make these distinctions clear:

- ***Mild to Moderate Fatigue (Routine)***: When fatigue occurs after activity and improves with rest or a meal, it's generally a normal "signal" for pacing. These episodes do not typically require medical intervention but should inform your plan for rest and gradual return to activity.

- ***"Red Flag" Fatigue Signals (Act Promptly)***: Be alert for fatigue that appears suddenly, is unusually severe, does not improve with rest, or is accompanied by other warning signs like shortness of breath, chest pain, difficulty swallowing, severe muscle weakness, confusion, or dizziness. These may signal an underlying medical complication, infection, medication reaction, or injury and require prompt medical review.

Table 3: Basic Decision Matrix Example

Fatigue Triggers and Characteristics	Recommended Response
Gradual onset, improves with rest, mild or moderate	Reduce pace, hydrate, monitor
Sudden onset, severe, with additional symptoms	Stop activity, notify caregiver or support, contact medical provider

Practical Tip:

Make this matrix visible—place a copy on the fridge or in your daily planner. Share it with anyone who regularly helps in your care. This can reduce uncertainty, increase confidence, and help avoid unnecessary risks.

Custom Fatigue Pattern Summary Table for Team Sharing

Once you've assembled a month or more of daily logs, weekly charts, and fatigue amplifier worksheets, the final step is consolidating this knowledge in an easy-to-understand summary. This summary will serve as a ready reference for your own adjustments and can be invaluable for care team members, new caregivers, or healthcare providers.

Structure your custom fatigue pattern summary with these elements:

- **Most Frequent Low-Energy Times**: *When do you consistently experience fatigue?*
- **Common Triggers**: *Which activities, environments, or emotions precipitate your symptoms most?*
- ***Notable "Red Flags"***: *What set of fatigue warnings have required attention in the past?*
- **Helpful Coping or Recovery Strategies**: *What actions have helped you rebound—structured rest, nutrition changes, specific medications, or environmental adjustments?*
- **Ongoing Questions or Concerns**: *Are there persistent patterns or "mystery symptoms" your care team should know about?*

Table 4: Sample Fatigue Pattern Summary Table

Time	Pattern
Morning (8-11am)	Moderate fatigue, worse after poorly slept nights; improves after breakfast and rest.
Afternoon (2-4pm)	Severe fatigue linked to meal skipping and standing work. Responds to hydration and short naps.
Evenings	Lowest fatigue, but anxious mood raises tiredness; needs quiet time.
Triggers	Hot weather, skipped meals, family stress, noise, overexertion.
Red Flags	Rapidly worsening fatigue with muscle weakness, twice required urgent evaluation.
Strategies	Scheduled snacks, reducing exposure to heat, daily relaxation exercises, consistent bedtime.

Sharing this table gives your team a clear window into your lived experience and supports more personalized care decisions. Remember to update it regularly as your patterns shift, or as you identify new triggers or effective interventions.

Taking Action: Your Fatigue Pattern Toolkit

Building an understanding of your fatigue patterns isn't a one-time project—it's an ongoing process that gets easier with practice and yields increasing rewards. Start by choosing tracking tools that fit your lifestyle and needs. Fill out your daily checklist, keep your weekly symptom chart in view, and regularly revisit your amplifiers worksheet and decision matrix. Each of these resources is a small act of self-advocacy—helping you reclaim agency in daily life and empowering those who support you to be more effective partners.

As you proceed through the chapters in this guide, the insights you gather here will help you personalize every recommendation, from meal scheduling to hydration protocols and snacking routines. You'll be equipped to make food and lifestyle choices that not only accommodate fatigue but actively work against its hold on your day.

If you feel overwhelmed, remember: even partial tracking—a few days' notes here, a summary table prepared before a doctor's visit—can be valuable. The information you gather is a foundation for better self-management, easier communication with your care team, and more hopeful, resilient living with PPS.

Energy-Balancing Meal Planning Framework (Systems)

Learning how to plan meals effectively is one of the most impactful steps you can take to support sustained energy and improved function when living with post-polio syndrome (PPS). While there is no universal formula, a tailored meal planning system can help offset unpredictable fatigue by providing your body with the right fuel at the right time. In this chapter, you'll find a practical, repeatable framework composed of simple templates, flexible rules, and real-world examples—all designed specifically for the unique nutritional needs and energy patterns of PPS.

The PPS Balanced Plate Template for Complete Nutrition

Meeting your energy needs with PPS goes well beyond counting calories. The goal is to assemble meals that not only supply sufficient macronutrients (protein, carbohydrates, and healthy fats) but also deliver the vitamins and minerals key to cellular energy production, muscle maintenance, and nervous system health. Research shows that people with PPS are at increased risk for deficiencies in vitamins B6, B12, folic acid, and iron—nutrients vital for combating fatigue and supporting muscle function.

The PPS Balanced Plate Template is a visual, portion-based system. Rather than focusing on precise measurements, you use your plate as a guide:

1. ***Fill ½ of your plate with non-starchy vegetables***. This includes leafy greens, broccoli, carrots, bell peppers, or cooked tomatoes. Vegetables provide dietary fiber (which aids digestion and helps prevent constipation, common in PPS) and deliver antioxidants and micronutrients like folate, magnesium, and vitamin C.
2. ***Allocate ¼ of your plate to lean protein sources***. These can be animal-based (skinless poultry, eggs, fish) or plant-based (tofu, beans, lentils). Protein is essential for muscle repair, reducing muscle breakdown, and supporting immune function—especially critical for those managing muscle weakness or loss after polio.
3. ***Set aside ¼ of your plate for energy-supporting carbohydrates***—think brown rice, quinoa, oats, sweet potatoes, or whole-grain bread. These foods provide slow-burning fuel to help maintain stable blood sugar and avert energy crashes. Choosing high-fiber, minimally processed options stabilizes energy levels

and supports heart health, which is important as inactivity can increase cardiovascular risk in PPS.

4. ***Add a small portion (about 1-2 tablespoons) of healthy fat***, such as olive oil, avocado, or nuts/seeds. Healthy fats supply essential fatty acids for cell health, help absorb fat-soluble vitamins (A, D, E, K), and contribute to a feeling of satisfaction after meals.

To round out your nutrient intake, aim to include a serving of an iron-rich food (such as lean red meat, beans, or spinach) or fortify meals with vitamin C-rich foods, which help increase iron absorption. For those with limited appetite or trouble eating, fortify foods with powdered milk, nut butters, or small amounts of oil to increase calories and nutrients without extra volume.

For people who rely on caregivers or need to simplify, pre-portioned ingredients or frozen mixed vegetables can streamline meal assembly while meeting nutritional needs.

Meal Timing and Spacing Ruleset

How and when you eat is just as important as what you eat for minimizing fatigue and keeping energy steady throughout the day. Many people with PPS experience post-meal crashes, where blood sugar plummets or digestion saps energy, especially if meals are too large or too far apart.

A nine-step meal timing and spacing ruleset can help optimize your eating schedule:

1. ***Aim for three main meals per day***, if possible, with one or two snacks, based on your typical appetite and symptom pattern.
2. ***Schedule meals and snacks*** at roughly the same time each day to regulate your body's internal clock and help prevent extreme hunger or overeating later.
3. ***Avoid very large meals*** that can overwhelm your digestion and cause energy dips.
4. ***Prioritize a balanced breakfast***—skipping breakfast can set up fatigue and low mood later in the day.
5. ***Space meals and snacks every 3-4 hours***, tailoring for when your personal fatigue tends to spike (for some people, spacing may be even shorter during high-fatigue cycles).
6. ***Pair carbohydrates with protein or healthy fat*** to slow digestion and prevent rapid changes in blood glucose.
7. ***Include hydration with meals***, but moderate large fluid intake during eating to prevent early fullness in those with small appetites or swallowing issues.
8. ***Listen to your body's cues***—if you notice low energy after eating, try reducing meal size and increasing meal frequency.
9. ***Use fatigue logs and symptom tracking*** to refine meal timing for when you have the most energy to prepare and eat your main meals.

By following these guidelines, you can preserve energy throughout your day, reduce the risk of post-meal slumps, and ensure that your nutritional intake is consistent despite appetite fluctuations or fatigue spikes.

Weekly Meal Grid Example: Adapting for Appetite and Simplicity

Fatigue and appetite are both highly variable in PPS, making one-size-fits-all meal plans impractical. Instead, a flexible Weekly Meal Grid offers an adaptable system that matches daily needs, energy, and ability to prepare food.

Here is a sample grid for a week, with options for both higher-energy days and periods of low appetite or extreme fatigue. The grid makes it easy to swap items between mealtimes or adjust portion sizes. On days when preparing a full meal is impossible, choose a simple "mini-meal" or snack box option.

Table 5: Weekly Meal Grid Example

	Breakfast	**Lunch**	**Dinner**	**Snack**
Mon	Scrambled eggs with sautéed spinach, whole-grain toast, orange slices	Chicken and vegetable soup with whole-grai n crackers	Baked salmon, roasted sweet potatoes, steamed broccoli	Greek yogurt with berries
Tue	Overnight oats with milk, chia	Turkey avocado	Lentil stew,	Apple slices with

	seeds, banana	wrap, carrot sticks	mixed green salad with pumpkin seeds	almond butter
Wed				
Thu				
Fri				
Sat				
Sun				

Low-Appetite Adaptation:

- ***Mini-meal***: Boiled egg, handful of grapes, cheese stick.
- ***Snack option***: Small smoothie with milk, fruit, and protein powder.

Apply this approach throughout the week: for higher-energy days, select more complex meals; for tough days, use pre-cooked freezer items, assemble snack plates, or rely on liquid meals like fortified soup or smoothies. The focus is flexibility—plan for easy modifications without sacrificing key nutrients.

Swap List: Energy-Boosting Foods vs. Common Fatiguing Triggers

Certain foods support steady energy, while others are more likely to trigger fatigue or digestive discomfort in PPS. Knowing the difference, and having a handy Swap List, can help you make quick decisions that fit your needs on any given day.

Energy-Boosting Swaps:

- ***Choose whole grains*** (quinoa, oats, brown rice) instead of refined grains (white rice, white bread), providing steadier energy and more fiber.
- ***Opt for lean proteins*** (fish, poultry, eggs, legumes) over high-fat or heavily processed meats; these are easier to digest and less likely to cause sluggishness.
- ***Use healthy oils*** (olive or canola) in small amounts rather than butter or shortening, to support heart health and muscle function.
- ***Select iron-rich plant foods*** (spinach, lentils) and combine with vitamin C sources (citrus, bell peppers) to combat or prevent iron deficiency anemia-linked fatigue.
- ***Incorporate nuts, seeds, and avocados*** for micronutrients and sustained satiety, in place of high-sugar snacks or pastries that may cause energy spikes and crashes.

Fatigue-Triggering Foods to Limit or Swap Out:

- ***Highly processed snacks*** (chips, cookies, packaged baked goods); replace with mixed nuts, roasted chickpeas, or fruit.
- ***Sugary beverages*** (soda, energy drinks); replace with water, herbal tea, or low-sugar electrolyte drinks.
- ***Fatty, fried foods***, which can slow digestion, worsen reflux, or trigger post-meal sleepiness; swap for baked or grilled options.
- ***Large amounts of caffeine***—moderate intake as excessive caffeine may disrupt sleep and amplify PPS fatigue.
- ***Overly salty foods***, which may worsen fluid retention for some individuals with PPS-related circulatory changes.

Keep in mind that PPS can affect individuals differently; if you notice a food consistently leads to greater fatigue, digestive upset, or other unwanted effects, use your fatigue and food log to fine-tune your personal Swap List.

Visual Meal Planning Board: Making Meal Choices Effortless

To put the meal planning system into daily action, a Visual Meal Planning Board can be a game-changer—especially when energy, memory, or attention are at a premium. The board serves as a central artifact for your fridge or kitchen wall, providing an at-a-glance guide to balanced choices and helping coordinate caregivers or family support.

How to Set Up Your Visual Board:

1. ***Print or handwrite your PPS Balanced Plate Template***, showing typical ingredients for each section of the plate, and laminate it for durability.
2. ***Create slots or magnets for breakfast, lunch, dinner, and snack options***, color-coded by complexity (green = easiest, yellow = moderate, red = high-effort). Place pre-prepared meal cards or photos in each slot.
3. ***Attach your Weekly Meal Grid***, updated at the beginning of each week. Include "high energy" vs. "low energy" options for each meal.
4. ***Add your personalized Swap List***—this helps quickly replace less optimal foods with PPS-friendly alternatives.
5. ***Post reminders*** about hydration, meal timing, and space for caregiver notes or special instructions—such as upcoming appointments or medication timing that affects meals.

For tech-friendly users, digital options such as meal-planning apps with customizable templates can be synced to smartphones or tablets. For those who prefer print, a simple paper chart protects focus and reduces decision fatigue.

Actionable Insights and Practical Examples

When building your meal planning system, focus on flexibility, simplicity, and personalization. If you have frequent periods of low appetite, prioritize nutrient-dense foods in small portions—think cottage cheese with fruit, fortified cereals, or nut-butter toast. To save time and energy, keep a rotating list of "core" meal and snack ideas on your Visual Meal Planning Board. Stock up on freezer and pantry staples that align with your balanced plate model.

For caregivers, involve those you support in selecting and adapting meals; this ensures dignity and autonomy while maintaining nutritional quality. If you ever notice patterns—such as repeated fatigue after specific meals, or persistent low energy at certain hours—use your logs and the meal planning framework to adjust meal composition or timing.

Remember: successful meal planning for PPS doesn't mean perfection or rigid rules. It means having a system in place that adapts to your reality, supports your best days, sustains you on the tougher ones, and puts you in charge of your energy—one balanced plate at a time.

Food Preparation Simplified for Low-Energy Days (Application)

Living with post-polio syndrome (PPS) means that energy is a precious, limited resource. Even basic food preparation can feel overwhelming on days when fatigue is at its peak. But regular, balanced meals are critical for stabilizing blood sugar, supporting muscle strength, and preventing further health complications. This chapter introduces practical, simplified strategies that transform kitchen routines into manageable, safe, and satisfying experiences—no matter how challenging your day may be.

Five-Minute Meal Assembly Checklist Using Pantry and Freezer Staples

On days when fatigue is highest, it's helpful to have a quick, reliable process for putting together nourishing meals without complicated steps or intensive cooking. A five-minute meal assembly checklist makes it possible to use pantry and freezer staples—food items that require little or no preparation but still meet your dietary needs. This is especially important for

PPS, where skipping meals or poor choices can lead to even greater weakness and delayed recovery.

Here's an easy-to-follow system:

1. **Choose a Protein:**
    - Canned beans or lentils (rinsed, low sodium)
    - Canned fish (tuna, salmon in water)
    - Pre-cooked frozen chicken strips or meatballs
    - Hard-boiled eggs (pre-cooked or purchased ready to eat)
    - Single-serve cottage cheese or Greek yogurt
2. **Pick a Whole Grain or Starch:**
    - Quick-cook oatmeal packets
    - Microwaveable brown rice or quinoa pouches
    - Whole grain crackers or rice cakes
    - Frozen diced sweet potatoes or peas
3. **Add a Fruit or Vegetable:**
    - Frozen mixed vegetables (steam-in-bag)
    - Canned no-salt-added green beans, carrots, or corn
    - Pre-washed salad greens
    - Applesauce or canned fruit in juice (not syrup)
4. **Enhance with Healthy Fats or Flavor:**
    - Olive oil drizzle or small handful of nuts

- Pre-sliced avocado or individual guacamole cups
- Shredded cheese (pre-packaged)

5. **Check Hydration and Add a Drink:**

   Water, herbal tea, low-sugar 100% juice box, or milk alternative

This assembly approach ensures you get a mix of protein, carbs, fat, and micronutrients without standing for long periods or using heavy cookware. Keep a printed copy of this checklist on your fridge for easy reminder and ask family or caregivers to help restock staples during grocery runs.

Adaptive Kitchen Tools Inventory for Safe, Low-Effort Food Prep

Safety and energy conservation in the kitchen start with the right equipment. PPS-related muscle weakness, joint pain, and limited mobility can make standard utensils difficult—raising the risk of falls, burns, or cuts. An adaptive kitchen tools inventory is a worthwhile investment that can empower independence and reduce unnecessary exertion.

Essential tools include:

- ***Long-Handled Reachers/Grabbers***: These extend your reach—for items in cabinets or the refrigerator—reducing the risk of stretching or climbing.

- ***Jar Openers and Electric Can Openers***: Arthritis-friendly, automatic models minimize grip strength and effort.
- ***Non-Slip Cutting Boards and Mats***: Secure surfaces that reduce movement and increase stability when slicing food.
- ***Adaptive Utensils***: Lightweight, easy-grip utensils with larger handles or built-in supports decrease hand fatigue.
- ***Pre-Cut and Ready-to-Eat Options***: Pre-diced vegetables, bagged salads, shredded cheese, and frozen prepared entrées save energy and reduce time spent handling knives or heavy pots.
- ***Microwave-Safe Dishes***: Sturdy, lightweight containers that eliminate the need for heavy or breakable cookware.
- ***Slow Cookers, Air Fryers, or Instant Pots***: These devices allow set-it-and-forget-it cooking, with automatic shut-offs and minimal manual handling.

Before making changes, review your kitchen and note which tasks feel hardest—then prioritize adaptive tools that directly address those challenges. Many local disability organizations or occupational therapists can offer advice or arrange trial sessions with select devices.

Batch Cooking and Freezing Planner: Identifying High-Energy Days and Aligning Meal Prep

Post-polio fatigue varies from day to day; honoring these rhythms helps keep meal routines sustainable. On high-energy days, use a batch cooking and freezing approach to prepare meals for future "down days." This method reduces overall effort, maximizes productive periods, and ensures you always have something nourishing on hand.

To create your batch cooking planner, follow these steps:

1. **Identify Patterns**

   Use your weekly fatigue log (see Table 1) to spot when you tend to have more energy—often mornings or the first half of the week.

2. **Choose Batch-Friendly Recipes**

   Soups, stews, casseroles, rice dishes, meatballs, chili, or sheet-pan roasted vegetables freeze and reheat well.

3. **Schedule Cooking in Short Intervals**

   Instead of a marathon kitchen session, break tasks into two or three short segments: chopping/prep, cooking, and portioning.

4. **Portion Before Freezing**

   Divide meals into single-serve containers. Label with contents and date for easy selection.

5. **Build a Freezer Inventory Sheet**

   List what's available and update as you use items. Post this list outside your freezer so you don't have to bend repeatedly or dig for options.

This planner allows you to always have at least several balanced, ready-to-eat meals when low energy strikes. If possible, involve family, caregivers, or friends for prep days, or use community resources (like Meals on Wheels or local post-polio support organizations) for assistance.

"No-Cook Nourishment" Emergency Snacks Table for Times of Peak Fatigue

There will be moments when even assembling a five-minute meal is too much. It's essential to maintain energy and avoid dehydration, especially since PPS can worsen with skipped meals or low blood sugar. Here is a list of emergency "no-cook" nourishment options—snacks that are safe, shelf-stable, and nutrient-rich for these situations.

No-Cook Nourishment Emergency Table:

- Nut Butter Pouches (single-serve, eaten with a spoon or spread on crackers)

- Trail Mix (nuts, seeds, dried fruit)
- Shelf-stable Protein Shake Boxes or Plant-Based Milk Drinks
- Whole Grain or Seed Crackers
- Unsweetened Applesauce Cups or Dried Fruit Packs
- Canned Beans (rinsed and eaten with minimal flavoring; use pop-top cans if grip is limited)
- Greek Yogurt or Cottage Cheese (pre-portioned, grab-and-go)
- Cheese Sticks or Babybel rounds
- Tuna or Salmon Pouches (pre-flavored, no draining needed)
- Cut Fruit Cups (packed in water or juice)

Place these foods in easy-to-reach spots (waist height, next to bed, or on accessible shelves) and check their expiry dates periodically. These options help keep your blood sugar steady and your energy levels from crashing, which is critical for preventing more profound fatigue or hospital visits.

Visual Portion Guide for Energy-Preserving Serving Sizes Specific to PPS

Eating more than you need can cause heaviness, post-meal fatigue, and digestive strain, while eating too little reduces fuel available for daily activity and muscle repair. For PPS, smaller, more frequent portions are often recommended to prevent energy crashes and make each meal or snack easier to manage physically. A visual approach to portion control side-steps the need for weighing or measuring food—saving you effort and frustration.

Visual Portion Guide for PPS:

- ***Protein*** (meat, beans, cheese): Palm-sized portion (about the size of a deck of playing cards)
- ***Carbohydrates*** (rice, pasta, potatoes, bread): Fist-sized serving (or half a standard cereal bowl)
- ***Vegetables***: Two cupped hands (about one heaping handful of leafy greens or steamed/microwaved veggies)
- ***Fruit***: Palm or handful (if whole fruit, about the size of a tennis ball)
- ***Healthy fats*** (nuts, oil, avocado): Thumb-sized (a tablespoon or small drizzle)

A sample balanced meal—using the five-minute checklist—might include a palm-sized portion of canned salmon, a fist-sized microwaveable pouch of quinoa, one cupped handful of frozen mixed vegetables microwaved, and a thumb-sized dollop of guacamole. This approach prevents overload and supports more stable, sustained energy.

Tips for Serving without Extra Effort:

- Use divided plates or bento-style lunchboxes to visualize the balance (protein, starch, vegetables) and avoid heavy pots.

- Portion directly from packages into bowls—no extra serving platters or utensils required.
- For snacks, pre-partition trail mix or dried fruit into resealable snack bags.

Putting It All Together: Everyday Examples

Maria, living with PPS, starts each week by noting her "good" and "bad" days in her symptom diary. On a Tuesday morning when she feels strongest, she makes two casseroles—eating one that night and freezing the rest in single-serve portions. She stocks her pantry with pop-top cans of beans, nut butter packets, and microwavable grains. On a day when walking feels like wading through mud, Maria skips the stove and pulls together a meal from her fridge: cottage cheese, whole wheat crackers, a cup of applesauce, and a handful of baby carrots. She uses a soft-grip fork and a plate with a rim to avoid spills. Maria's daughter, when visiting, helps her update a snack bin at eye-level with protein shakes, cut fruit, and portioned nuts. With these simple adaptations and routines, Maria feels confident she can manage her nutrition—even when her body and energy disagree.

Getting Support and Building Routines

While the goal is greater independence, it's not a failure to ask for help—or to use shortcuts. Share your food prep plan with caregivers or family so they know how to assist or shop for your "low-energy day" foods. Many local organizations for people with physical disabilities offer resources, adaptive cooking classes, or kitchen tool lending programs. By committing to small, realistic adjustments now, you can reduce daily stress and protect your functional capacity in the long term.

Adapting Kitchens and Attitudes

Simplifying food preparation is not about giving up "home-cooked" meals or settling for unsatisfying options—it's a shift in perspective. Every adaptation, from microwaveable soups to pre-washed greens, is a purposeful strategy in preserving energy for what matters most to you. With the right planning, a supportive environment, and a willingness to embrace new tools, eating well with PPS is possible even on your hardest days.

Hydration and Electrolyte Protocols (Execution)

For individuals living with post-polio syndrome (PPS), hydration is far more than a simple daily health tip: it is a critical piece in the puzzle of managing energy, decreasing fatigue, and minimizing secondary complications. Yet, for many, mobility and swallowing challenges introduce very real barriers to consistent hydration. This chapter delivers actionable systems for tracking hydration, balancing electrolytes, and coordinating support—all tailored for the realities of PPS.

Daily Hydration Tracking Sheet Tailored for Mobility Constraints and Swallowing Issues

Fatigue, muscle weakness, and swallowing difficulties (dysphagia) common in PPS can make it hard to remember, reach, or ingest fluids throughout the day. While dehydration increases risks of muscle cramps, constipation, urinary complications, and even confusion, over-hydration—especially if kidney or cardiac issues are present—can lead to swelling and breathing problems. Precision and personalization are key for safe hydration.

A Daily Hydration Tracking Sheet offers a structured, visual way to help you (or your caregiver) log fluid intake, track progress, and spot patterns that need attention. When building or using a tracking sheet as a PPS survivor:

- Choose your preferred unit (milliliters, fluid ounces, cups) and establish your daily hydration goal in partnership with your clinician or registered dietitian, since needs may vary based on kidney, heart, or swallowing function.
- Use printed sheets, a large-print notepad, or a simple digital device with reminders—opt for the tool you can most easily access given your grip strength and visual needs.
- Adapt entries to include all sources of fluids, not just water. For those with dysphagia, include thicker liquids, broth, or hydrating foods like gelatin, yogurt, or blended soups that are easier to swallow.
- Break the day into manageable time slots (for example: wake-up, morning, lunch, afternoon, dinner, evening) to prompt regular sips and give multiple "small win" goals instead of one big, overwhelming quota.

Consider these sample tracking columns:

Table 6: Sample Daily Hydration Tracking Sheet

Time of day	What and how much was consumed	Swallowing ease rating (easy, moderate, difficult)	Comments (cramping, fatigue, fullness, or difficulties noted)

For caregivers, leave space to initial or check off when assistance was provided. This ensures accountability and continuity, especially if care is shared among multiple people.

By using this tracking sheet every day, you'll quickly develop an accurate picture of how much liquid you're really getting, how fluid intake affects your symptoms, and where adaptive strategies might be needed to make hydration more achievable.

Electrolyte-Balancing Drink Recipes and Their Role in Managing PPS-Related Weakness or Cramping

Alongside water, the body depends on electrolytes—minerals such as sodium, potassium, calcium, and magnesium—to regulate muscle function, heart rhythm, and nerve impulses. For PPS survivors, imbalance can show up as muscle cramps, pronounced fatigue, or sudden weakness, particularly after sweating, during illness, or when diuretics (medications that increase urine output) are prescribed.

Ready-to-drink electrolyte solutions and sports drinks can be useful but are often high in sugar or sodium, which is not ideal for those managing weight, cardiac, or blood pressure concerns. Instead, consider homemade, low-sugar recipes that offer better control over your intake:

Simple PPS-Friendly Electrolyte Drink Recipe

Ingredients:

- 2 cups clean water (use warm or room temperature for easier swallowing)
- ¼ cup 100% orange juice (for potassium and subtle sweetness)
- ¼ tsp salt (for sodium; adjust down if you are on a sodium-restricted diet—check with your clinician first)
- 1 tbsp honey or a sugar substitute (for flavor)
- Optional: a splash of coconut water (for additional potassium and magnesium) if not contraindicated

Instructions:

1. Stir thoroughly.
2. This can be sipped slowly throughout the day or offered during meals for easier swallowing.

Vary juice types (such as diluted apple or grape juice) to prevent flavor boredom or irritation if you have oral sensitivity.

If swallowing is a challenge, consult a speech-language pathologist about thickening agents, which can be added to these drinks to ensure safe swallowing without reducing their hydrating effect.

Use these drinks when you notice muscle cramps, after periods of sweating (such as after physical therapy or hot weather), or as part of your daily routine if you have a history of electrolyte disturbances. If you experience persistent symptoms—new weakness, irregular heartbeat, or confusion—seek prompt medical advice for possible bloodwork and further adjustment of your protocol.

Water Bottle Placement Plan to Ensure Access in Key Home or Work Areas

Planning where and how you'll access water dramatically improves the odds of meeting daily hydration targets, especially when mobility is reduced or arm weakness is present.

A Water Bottle Placement Plan involves assessing your routines and physically staging bottles or cups where you spend the most time:

- Place lightweight, easy-to-grip water bottles or cups at your bedside, near your favorite chair, and by your workspace (desk or table) for effortless access.

- Choose bottles with spouts, straws, or handles that are simple to open and hold, considering grip strength and coordination.
- Keep a bottle within arm's reach on your mobility device (walker, wheelchair, or scooter), using commercial cup holders, carabiners, or even Velcro straps.
- For those who forget to refill, use bottles with volume markers to track how much you're drinking, and ask family or caregivers to check/refill at scheduled times (such as meal or medication times).
- Store extra, prefilled bottles in the fridge or a cooler, so you don't need to walk or wheel to the kitchen for every refill—especially helpful overnight or when fatigued.
- Don't forget high-traffic or "pause" points: the entryway, bathroom counter, medication caddy, or hobby/work corners. If you use adaptive trays or reachers, ensure your bottles are compatible for easy transfer and opening.

The goal: Eliminate as many barriers as possible between you and your next sip. Simple, visible reminders are especially helpful for those with memory challenges or fluctuating fatigue.

Signs of Over-Hydration Versus Dehydration: PPS Pocket Guide

Knowing what to look for keeps you safe from both too little and too much fluid intake—a real consideration for individuals with chronic health conditions, mobility challenges, or impaired thirst drive.

Use this easy PPS Pocket Guide to recognize early warning signs:

1. **Classic Dehydration Signs:**
    - Dry mouth, thick saliva
    - Dark-colored, concentrated urine (or urinating less often)
    - Headache or dizziness, especially when standing up
    - Muscle cramps or sudden fatigue
    - Fast heart rate
    - Constipation
    - Sunken eyes or feeling confused
2. **Classic Over-Hydration Signs:**
    - Swelling in feet, ankles, or hands
    - Sudden weight gain (1–2 pounds or more in 1–2 days)
    - Puffiness around face or eyelids
    - Shortness of breath, especially lying down

- Frequent urination (clear, almost colorless urine every hour)
- Nausea, headache, or confusion (in severe cases)
- Persistent cough, especially alongside swelling

With PPS, dehydration may worsen fatigue, increase cramping, and contribute to difficulties with bowel and bladder management. Over-hydration is usually a concern for those with underlying kidney, heart, or hormonal issues, and may exacerbate swelling or breathing difficulties.

Carry this "pocket" checklist or post it on your fridge. If you spot signs of dehydration, increase fluid intake gradually unless you have medical restrictions. If symptoms of over-hydration develop, contact your care team right away—especially if you experience swelling, breathing difficulty, or rapid weight change.

When in doubt, track symptoms alongside your hydration sheet and share patterns with your doctor or nurse. Always follow fluid restrictions set by your clinicians—never increase or decrease fluids abruptly without medical input.

"Hydration Partner" Checklist for Caregiver or Family Coordination

Hydration is more than an individual task; for many with PPS, involving a trusted caregiver or family member makes protocols safer and more sustainable. A "Hydration Partner" checklist formalizes roles, improves consistency, and fosters shared accountability.

Hydration Partner Checklist:

Daily Routine Checks:

- ☐ Review the personalized daily hydration goal and tracking sheet together every morning.
- ☐ Confirm access to safe, preferred fluids in all main living areas (bedroom, bathroom, living room, kitchen/work area).
- ☐ Ensure adaptive cups/bottles are clean and ready.

Scheduled Refill/Assistance:

- ☐ Identify three to five specific time windows to prompt refills, offer drinks, or remind you (such as after meals, medication times, before therapy, and bedtime).
- ☐ Prepare and label electrolyte drinks ahead of time if needed.

Swallowing Safety:

- Observe for coughing, difficulty swallowing, or changes in voice during or after sips—if noted, alert a speech-language pathologist or care provider.
- Use appropriate thickening agents as directed.

Symptom Monitoring:

- ☐ Review the Dehydration/Over-hydration Pocket Guide daily for signs of imbalance.
- ☐ Log any concerning symptoms (headache, swelling, new fatigue, or confusion) for discussion.

Coordination and Communication:

- ☐ Mark off completed items on the hydration tracking sheet (digital or paper).
- ☐ Communicate with other family members or aides about daily progress, needs, and any changes in routine.
- ☐ Adjust placement of bottles or drinks based on daily activity (for example: move a bedside cup to a wheelchair on therapy days).

Weekly Review:

At the end of each week, review intake and symptom patterns, and adjust protocols with input from clinical professionals as needed.

For caregivers, this checklist reduces cognitive load—you know exactly what steps to follow, and your loved one feels confident hydration won't be forgotten. For those living alone, consider asking a friend or neighbor to check in regularly, or use reminder apps with designated emergency contacts if symptoms emerge.

Final Thoughts

Hydration and electrolyte balance, while seemingly simple, are central to sustaining post-polio function, minimizing fatigue, and supporting independence day-to-day. By layering together personalized tracking, practical placement, balanced recipes, and clear support systems, you create a fail-safe structure robust enough to weather the unpredictable waves of PPS.

Use these protocols as a living toolkit: refine, adapt, and adjust them as your needs, abilities, and living situation change. Involve your care team early and share your progress—they may uncover new ways to fine-tune your plan for even greater ease and effectiveness.

With the right daily practices and the support of your Hydration Partner, you move one step closer to steady energy, safer routines, and maximized quality of life.

Strategic Snacking: Sustaining Energy Between Meals (Tools)

For individuals with post-polio syndrome (PPS), managing energy is not just about what you eat at mealtimes—it's about ensuring a steady supply of usable fuel throughout the day. Many people living with PPS experience pronounced fatigue, post-meal sluggishness, and difficulty recovering from energy dips if meals are too far apart. Strategic snacking becomes an essential tool for keeping energy levels even, minimizing sudden lows, and improving daily function. In this chapter, you'll discover practical resources to make snack time supportive, safe, and truly sustaining for those with PPS.

Energy Sustain Snack List: Optimized for Slow Release and Ease of Eating

Choosing snacks that deliver slow, consistent energy—without spiking blood sugar or causing digestive discomfort—is especially important for people with PPS. Fatigue and muscle weakness can make handling, chewing, and swallowing certain foods difficult. For this reason, the focus should be on foods that require minimal effort to eat but still provide lasting energy.

Below is a curated list of "Energy Sustain" snacks that are easy to prepare, gentle on digestion, and suitable for those with chewing or swallowing challenges:

- ***Smooth Nut Butters (peanut, almond, sunflower) on soft whole grain bread or crackers***: These provide complex carbohydrates and healthy fats, releasing energy steadily over time, and can be spread thick or thin according to ease of swallowing.
- ***Low-sugar Greek yogurt or cottage cheese***: Offers protein and some fat to satiate and slow the release of sugars, and can be blended with soft fruits like bananas or peaches for extra nutrition.
- ***Soft-cooked oatmeal with ground flaxseed and soft fruits***: Oats digest slowly, delivering steady fuel, while flaxseed adds omega-3s for joint and nerve health.
- ***Hummus or bean dip with soft pita or thin rice cakes***: Beans are a great source of protein and fiber, and hummus is smooth enough for those with mild swallowing concerns.

Chia pudding made with milk or dairy alternatives: Chia seeds swell and soften, offering a nutrient-dense option that is easy to swallow and can be flavored with vanilla or cinnamon for variety.

- ***Applesauce with a sprinkle of cinnamon and chopped nuts (if tolerated)***: Offers simple carbs but can be balanced with ground flax, chia, or soft nut butters.
- ***Mashed avocado with soft cheese on thin, soft whole grain toast***: Avocado provides healthy fats and vitamins with a creamy texture.
- ***Soft-boiled or scrambled eggs***: These are easy to chew and swallow, deliver complete protein, and can be seasoned lightly.
- ***Homemade trail mix with chopped soft dried fruit and small seeds (such as shelled sunflower seeds), omitting hard, whole nuts for easier chewing***: Choose low-sugar dried fruits to avoid energy spikes.

These snacks are designed to avoid causing blood sugar spikes which can contribute to both sudden fatigue and longer-term metabolic issues, all while being mindful of the swallowing and chewing needs common in PPS.

Snack Placement Matrix: Strategic Stocking Across Daily Environments

To maximize the benefit of strategic snacking, placement matters just as much as selection. Mobility limitations can make frequent trips to the kitchen taxing or even unsafe, so integrating snacks into key locations in your routine is essential.

Consider the following Snack Placement Matrix to keep sustaining snacks within safe, effortless reach:

1. **Bedside Table**
    - Store individually wrapped soft granola bars, squeeze packs of nut butter, applesauce cups, or ready-to-drink protein shakes.
    - Place snacks in a small, easy-open basket or container that doesn't require two hands to access.
    - For those with swallowing issues, keep water or a beverage thickener alongside for safe swallowing.

2. **Work or Activity Area**
    - Use a small desktop bin or soft cooler bag for perishable snacks.
    - Stock with items like low-sugar yogurt tubs, soft fruit cups, or cut vegetables with dip.
    - Place this kit at a level that avoids bending or reaching—ideally on the same level as your workspace.

3. **Mobility Bags or Wheelchair Attachments**
    - Use pocket-sized, easy-open packs of nut butters, soft protein bars, or resealable pouches of trail mix.

- Choose packaging with large tabs or notches to accommodate limited grip strength.
- Avoid snacks that crumble or spill easily during transport for safety and cleanliness.

4. **TV or Reading Area**
   - Use a small caddy to store pre-portioned snacks such as oatmeal raisin bites, soft baked bars, or squeeze yogurts.
   - Keep a napkin and spoon close by for cleanliness and easy eating.

5. **Car or On-the-Go**
   - Choose shelf-stable, non-melting snacks like soft fig bars, applesauce pouches, or vacuum-sealed protein shakes.
   - Replace these regularly to ensure freshness.

A written checklist of daily snack locations encourages routine restocking and prevents accidental omission, especially on high-fatigue days. For those with a caregiver, this list can be part of a shared care plan to ensure snacks are always within reach.

Prep-Ahead Snack Storage Guide: Ensuring Safety and Freshness

Food safety is vital, especially when snacks are stored at room temperature or carried throughout the day. Improper storage can lead to spoilage and increase the risk of foodborne illness—risks that may affect PPS patients more severely due to compromised immunity or slower response time to symptoms.

Here's how to store common snacks safely:

1. **Room Temperature (up to 8–12 hours):**
    - Shelf-stable items like granola bars, nut butter squeeze packs, unopened applesauce cups, and sealed trail mix are safe.
    - Avoid perishable dairy, eggs, or soft cheeses outside a cold pack for long periods.
2. **Refrigerated Storage (up to 3–5 days):**
    - Yogurts, soft cheeses, hummus, cut fruits, and chia pudding should be stored in the fridge between 34°F and 40°F (1°C to 4°C).
    - Use small, single-serving containers to minimize handling and reduce contamination risk.
3. **Freezer (up to 2–3 months):**
    - Some snacks like certain muffins, soft granola bites, or banana-based treats can be frozen and thawed overnight.
    - Always label containers with date and contents. Discard any items with signs of freezer burn or changed texture after thawing.

4. **Coolers or Insulated Pouches:**

   When traveling or during extended outings, keep perishable snacks chilled with ice packs, aiming to consume them within four hours.

5. **Extra tips:**
   - Use clear storage bins or color-coded lids to match snacks with required temperature zones.
   - Check use-by dates weekly, especially on individually packaged snacks for quick-grab safety.
   - For those with swallowing challenges, avoid snacks with small, hard pieces that may become harder with time (like aging muffins or over-dried fruit).

Snack Frequency and Portion Control Ruleset

Snacking offers the greatest benefit for PPS when done consistently but not excessively. Large, frequent snacks can lead to digestive fatigue, weight gain, and even sleep disturbance if consumed too close to bedtime.

Follow these guidelines to achieve optimal energy support:

1. **Timing:**
    - Aim for a snack every 2½ to 3½ hours between main meals, but not within one hour of bedtime to prevent reflux or interrupted sleep.
    - For individuals prone to early fatigue, an additional snack in the afternoon can prevent pre-meal energy drops.
    - If you wake at night hungry, consult with your clinician about adjusting meal timing rather than adding a late-night snack.
2. **Portion Size:**
    - Use a visual guide: a snack should fit into the palm of your hand or be the size of a tennis ball.
    - Focus on 100–200 calorie servings to prevent excess calorie intake while providing enough fuel to bridge to the next meal.
    - Measure or pre-portion snacks at the start of the week to avoid mindless overeating, especially with grab-and-go items.
3. **Digestive Fatigue Management:**
    - Choose snacks that are moist and easy to chew—dry, hard, or fibrous foods can be taxing.
    - Alternate between different snack types through the week for digestive variety.
    - A simple snack log or use of a kitchen timer/reminder app can support consistent but

appropriate intake, reducing both the risk of fatigue spikes and nighttime waking.

"Snack Swap" Decision Table: Adapting Snacks for Dietary Restrictions

Many living with PPS also manage secondary health conditions—like high blood pressure, diabetes, or cholesterol issues—that require dietary limits. Fortunately, strategic swaps can maintain the energy-sustaining benefits of snacks while meeting individual health criteria.

Below is a decision table for common snack adaptations:

Table 7: "Snack Swap" Decision Table

Restriction	Original Snack Idea	Adapted Snack Option	Notes
Low Sodium	Cheese and whole grain crackers	Low-sodium cottage cheese & unsalted rice cakes	Choose fresh, low-salt cheese
Low Sugar/ Diabetes	Granola bar with dried fruit	Nut butter on thin apple slices	Use unsweetened nut butter
Gluten-Free	Oatmeal raisin muffin	Gluten-free oat/flax muffin	Double-check oats are certified
Dairy-Free	Greek yogurt with soft fruit	Coconut/soy yogurt + chia seeds	Choose unflavored, low-sugar
Nut Allergy	Almond butter & banana on toast	Sunflower seed butter & banana	Verify allergy friendly brands
Easy Swallowing	Trail mix with seeds and nuts	Smooth applesauce with flax/chia	Avoid hard, chewy textures

High Protein	Rice cake with soft cheese	Rice cake with mashed chickpeas + tahini	Adds fiber, protein

When planning snack swaps:

1. Always read ingredient lists for allergens and avoid added sugars and excess sodium, especially in pre-made options.
2. Use the nutrition facts panel to compare choices; aim for snacks with less than 6g sugar and under 120mg sodium whenever possible for those with restrictions.
3. If homemade, choose recipes that allow easy modification—swap regular flour for a gluten-free blend, or cow's milk for fortified soy milk.

Practical Tips in Action

Let's say Jane, a woman living with PPS, notices a mid-morning dip in her energy that makes it hard to focus or complete light chores. By keeping a small caddy of soft granola bites and applesauce near her favorite chair, she can refuel without struggling to the kitchen. On days when her appetite is low but she needs protein, she swaps in individual tubs of low-sugar Greek yogurt, stored in a desk-side cooler with an ice pack. When her doctor advises lowering her salt intake, she shifts to unsalted rice cakes with avocado spread, maintaining energy balance but meeting her health needs.

Small, strategic changes like these can transform the role snacks play in the daily life of someone with PPS—lifting energy, improving alertness, and supporting safe, independent living.

Pantry, Fridge, and Freezer Organization (Execution)

For people living with post-polio syndrome (PPS), navigating the kitchen is often a daily exercise in balancing basic nourishment with safety and energy preservation. Routine activities like reaching for food, bending to retrieve ingredients, and sorting through crowded shelves are not just inconvenient—they come with an increased risk of falls, injury, or fatigue that can derail an entire day's plan. Successful meal preparation, snack assembly, and even hydration are intricately linked to how your kitchen spaces are laid out and managed. In this chapter, you'll find a targeted, practical approach to organizing the pantry, fridge, and freezer with the unique needs of PPS in mind—transforming your kitchen from a potential obstacle course into a supportive hub for independence and well-being.

Accessible Storage System Layout for Minimizing Reaching, Bending, and Risk of Falls

The effects of PPS—muscle weakness, reduced range of motion, and heightened fatigue—mean that traditional kitchen layouts aren't always practical. Repeated reaching overhead or bending low can increase the likelihood of falls or muscular overuse, compromising safety and contributing to further energy depletion. Adapting your food storage strategy can significantly reduce these risks and make daily food-related tasks both safe and sustainable.

Prioritize frequently used items at waist-to-shoulder height. Store daily essentials such as whole grains, canned vegetables, and go-to condiments on shelves that fall between the hips and the eyes when you're standing or sitting. This range minimizes the need to stretch upward or crouch downward—two movements that can be taxing and dangerous for those with PPS.

Reserve low or high shelves for light or infrequently accessed goods. Place lighter, seldom-used foods (like extras of dry pasta or seasonal baking supplies) on higher or lower shelves, but ensure they're not in heavy containers. Avoid storing any heavy or bulky items above shoulder height or near the floor, as retrieving them can strain weakened muscles and compromise balance.

Use pull-out drawers, lazy susans, or bins for deeper shelves. Clear bins or lazy susans make it easier to see and reach foods stored in the back without bending, twisting, or needing help. Pull-out shelves minimize overexertion and allow for a more organized view of available ingredients.

For those using mobility aids or who have difficulty standing for longer periods, consider:

- A wheeled kitchen cart that can serve as both a prep area and a portable storage solution, especially for commonly used items.
- Wall-mounted, easy-grip handles near storage areas for stability.
- Plaques or labels in large font for identifying foods by touch or glance.

If available, enlist a family member, friend, or caregiver to help arrange and maintain the layout. Periodically review the setup to ensure it continues meeting your needs as your condition evolves.

"Essential Foods Only" Restocking Checklist for Predictably Nutritious Options

Stocking the right foods—while avoiding food clutter—lays the groundwork for predictable, balanced eating with less decision fatigue. For people with PPS, it is critical to keep shelves filled with truly essential, nutritious options, minimizing food waste and temptation to reach for less beneficial choices.

A core restocking checklist should cover the following categories, focusing on nutrient density, ease of preparation, and energy efficiency:

- ☐ ***Lean protein sources***: Canned tuna or salmon (in water), rotisserie chicken, eggs, and pre-portioned cooked legumes (such as lentils or chickpeas).
- ☐ ***High-fiber carbohydrates***: Brown rice, whole-grain bread, oats, and low-sugar cereals.
- ☐ ***Shelf-stable produce***: Canned tomatoes (no salt added), canned or boxed beans, unsweetened applesauce, and low-sodium vegetable soups.
- ☐ ***Healthy fats***: Olive oil, peanut or almond butter, mixed nuts, or individual packets of seeds.
- ☐ ***Easy-access dairy or dairy alternatives***: Individual Greek yogurt cups, cheese sticks, shelf-stable plant milks.
- ☐ ***Frozen vegetables and fruits***: Mixed vegetable blends, spinach, berries, or smoothie blends, chosen for no added sugars or sauces.
- ☐ ***Hydration***: Bottled water, low-sugar electrolyte drinks, caffeine-free herbal teas, and broths.
- ☐ ***Emergency energy items***: Nutrition bars with balanced protein and carbohydrates (check food label for "complete" protein and low added sugar).

This list can be customized to your preferences and dietary needs. The goal is to maintain a concise, manageable inventory that supports consistent meal assembly and snack choices without overburdening your storage space or your energy.

Shelf-Level Sorting Map for Prioritizing Easy-to-Reach, Energy-Optimized Ingredients

Once you've narrowed your inventory to essentials, group foods within each storage area to optimize access and minimize fatigue:

1. ***Eye-level shelves***: Stock ready-to-eat or frequently used ingredients—nutritional shakes, portioned snacks, sandwich fixings, and single-serve fruits.

2. ***Waist-level shelves***: Place medium-weight foods such as canned goods, grains, and jars of spreads—these are easy to slide or lift without effort and offer daily variety.

3. ***Lower shelves (if reachable without risk)***: Store lightweight staples or multiples (like extra rolls of paper towels), never essentials.

4. ***In the fridge***: Assign a designated "first grab" area to items for quick meals (yogurts, single-serve vegetables, boiled eggs, pre-washed salad greens).

Keep leftovers in clear, labeled containers at the front, not in the back where they're hard to reach or see.

5. ***In the freezer***: Stand upright pre-cut vegetable bags and single-meal frozen entrees on the top shelf, laying heavier or infrequently used items below. Always avoid crouching or using step stools—if you require assistance for lower shelves, communicate this clearly with caregivers or family.

Use labels or color-coding systems to quickly identify what's inside and when it should be used. For example, red stickers for "use this week," yellow for "soon," and green for "stock/backups."

Backup Food Supply Kit for Days When Shopping is Not Possible

Unpredictable fatigue spikes, bad weather, or transportation challenges can sometimes make leaving home for groceries impossible. Creating a small but mighty backup food kit helps keep you nourished and safe during unforeseen disruptions.

Your kit should include:

1. Shelf-stable, easy-to-open entrées (e.g., pull-top canned soups or heat-and-eat meals).
2. Ready-to-drink meal supplements or shakes.
3. Nut butter squeeze packs with whole-grain crackers.

4. Individual fruit cups (packed in water or juice, not syrup) or small boxes of raisins or dried fruit.
5. Vacuum-sealed tuna or chicken salad kits with utensils.
6. Electrolyte packets for mixing with water, especially important if weakness or dehydration may occur.
7. Bottled water, enough for at least three days (aim for at least one quart per person per day).
8. List of local takeout restaurants or meal delivery services offering reliable, nutrition-conscious options.

Store your backup kit together in a clearly labeled, accessible location, ideally at waist height near the kitchen entrance or adjacent to the refrigerator. Rotate the kit at least twice a year, checking for expiry and replacing items as needed. Let household members and caregivers know the kit's location and intended use.

Food Expiry and Waste Minimization Tracker to Reduce Food Spoilage and Overexertion

Proper tracking systems are crucial for reducing two major risks: food waste (which wastes money and energy) and accidental foodborne illness (which can be medically risky for people with chronic conditions like PPS). A good tracker eliminates the need for repeated bending to hunt for dates or guess at safe-use windows.

Set up a basic system:

1. Record new purchase dates and "use by" deadlines for all perishable food items. A simple dry-erase board posted on the fridge or a notepad on a nearby countertop works well.

2. For leftovers or prepared meals, use removable labels on containers to note when they were prepared and their "eat by" dates.

3. Practice a "first-in, first-out" rule—always bring older foods to the front and place newly purchased goods toward the back, ensuring nothing is forgotten until spoiled.

4. Once per week (or during shopping/prep cycles), review the board/list to prioritize what needs to be eaten first, then plan snack and meal choices accordingly.

If you have support from a caregiver or family member, make food expiry tracking part of the weekly routine, and delegate disposal of outdated items to avoid unnecessary bending or reaching.

Tracking expiry not only preserves safety but helps conserve valuable energy. By limiting the time spent sorting through cluttered shelves, people with PPS can reduce their risk of fatigue and devote their efforts to more meaningful routines.

Practical Example: Sarah's Accessible Kitchen

Sarah, a 65-year-old PPS survivor, found that traditional deep pantry shelves made snack and ingredient retrieval a major source of frustration and fatigue. Working with her daughter, she reorganized her kitchen so that all daily-use foods (including canned beans, whole-grain tortillas, peanut butter, and nutritional shakes) sat at chest height in see-through bins on slide-out shelves.

Her fridge now boasts a top-shelf "Quick Meals" box with pre-cut fruit, yogurt cups, and individually wrapped cheese sticks. A dry-erase magnet board tracks expiration dates and a backup kit in a brightly labeled plastic tub contains three days' worth of ready-to-eat foods and meals. Sarah rarely throws away spoiled food, spends less time in the kitchen, and feels more independent, relying only on minimal help with shelf restocking every few weeks.

Actionable Insights for Immediate Organization

- ***Conduct a shelf audit***: Remove all items, assess for frequency of use, and categorize foods as "daily essential," "occasional," or "backup."

- ***Relocate essentials***: Place all "daily essential" foods within easy arm's reach, between waist and shoulder height.
- ***Set up your tracking system***: Start a dry-erase expiry board and label leftovers and perishables.

Assemble your backup food kit, and establish a reminder (calendar or phone alert) to check its contents twice yearly.

Communicate your storage system with all who help you at home; consistent routines prevent confusion and keep your space predictable, safe, and efficient.

By investing thoughtful time in the initial setup and keeping systems simple and consistent, you'll spend less energy on routine tasks and more on the things that matter most to you—whether that's enjoying meals, connecting with loved ones, or simply getting through the day with greater ease.

Food First, Medication Second: Managing Nutrient-Drug Interactions (Mechanisms)

Managing post-polio syndrome (PPS) fatigue and other symptoms often involves a mix of medications and dietary adjustments. Yet, what many don't realize is how closely food and drugs interact—sometimes working together, sometimes counteracting each other, and sometimes even creating new side effects. For individuals with PPS and their caregivers, understanding these interactions is an essential step in making daily routines safer, more effective, and less overwhelming. Knowing which foods can enhance or diminish medication effects, when to eat around dosing, and how to spot warning signs allows you to place food at the center of your management plan—relegating medication to its appropriate, supportive role.

Table of Common PPS Medications and Their Key Food Interactions

A first step in practical symptom management is learning which medications are commonly used in PPS care and how food can help or hinder their action. The following table summarizes some typical medications prescribed for PPS, along with essential food-interaction notes. Always refer to your specific prescription and check with your pharmacist, since individual variations and new recommendations do occur.

Table 8: Common PPS Medications and Key Food Interactions

Common PPS Medication	Primary Use	Key Food Interactions
Acetaminophen (Tylenol)	Pain relief	Nearly always safe with or without food; taking with food may reduce stomach upset in sensitive individuals.
Non-Steroidal Anti-Inflammatory Drugs (NSAIDs, e.g., ibuprofen)	Pain and inflammation	Recommended to take with food to reduce risk of stomach irritation or ulceration; avoid alcohol and excessive caffeine, which increase GI risks.
Antidepressants (e.g., tricyclics, SSRIs)	Depression, sleep, and pain management	Some should be taken with food to reduce GI upset; avoid foods containing tyramine with certain older antidepressants, as this can cause dangerous blood pressure spikes
Muscle relaxants (e.g., baclofen)	Muscle pain or spasm	Take with meals or snacks to lessen drowsiness and stomach upset. Alcohol, excessive caffeine, and sedating foods should be

		limited.
Statins and other cholesterol-lowering agents	Heart disease risk mitigation	Some, like simvastatin, are best taken in the evening and should avoid grapefruit, which increases side effects risk.
Corticosteroids (if prescribed for inflammation)	Inflammation and pain	Often best taken with meals to decrease risk of GI irritation; may increase appetite, so balanced meal planning is key.
Vitamin D, calcium, or multivitamin supplements	Bone health, general nutrition	Take with food to increase absorption (except for iron, see below). Avoid taking with high-oxalate foods when possible as these can lower benefit.
Iron supplements	Anemia, energy support	Optimal absorption on an empty stomach, but often causes stomach upset—taking with a small fruit or juice high in vitamin C is beneficial, but avoid dairy/calcium-rich foods within two hours as they block iron absorption.

If any of these categories or examples sound unfamiliar, review your medication labels and ask your pharmacist for updated, simplified interaction guidance—especially if you take generics or combination products.

Meal Timing Grid for Optimal Absorption of Medications Taken With or Without Food

Matching meal and medication schedules can minimize side effects and maximize treatment benefits. Use this straightforward grid to plan when to take common PPS medications based on typical absorption patterns and digestive comfort:

Table 9: Meal Timing Sample

Take with Food	• NSAIDs • Corticosteroids • Muscle relaxants • Many antidepressants	Schedule these doses right after, or at the end of, your main meal or a substantial snack. Taking alongside protein, whole grains, or a little healthy fat can further ease digestion.
Take on an Empty Stomach	• Iron supplements (unless intolerable) • Some thyroid medications • Selected painkillers	Try to wait at least one hour before or two hours after meals. For iron, a small glass of orange juice can boost uptake; avoid coffee, milk, tea, or high-fiber foods during this window to prevent absorption block.
Flexible—With or Without Food	• Acetaminophen • Most vitamin or mineral supplements (except iron)	Assess personal tolerance; if you notice stomach upset, shift to mealtime dosing.
Special Timing	• Statins (some best at night) • Certain drugs that should not be taken with high-fat or grapefruit-containing foods	Carefully read prescription instructions and ask your pharmacist about any time-of-day or food-specific considerations.

A daily chart or calendar reminder, or using a simple paper grid taped to the medicine cabinet, can help keep meal and medication schedules aligned while minimizing confusion and missed doses.

"Alert Foods" List: Identifying Items That May Diminish or Enhance Drug Efficacy

Certain foods can dramatically change how well (or poorly) your body uses specific medications. For people with PPS, who may rely on a delicate mix of drugs to manage symptoms, these "alert foods" deserve extra attention in daily meal planning:

- ***High-calcium foods (milk, cheese, yogurt)***: Interfere with iron absorption, and sometimes with certain antibiotics or thyroid medications.
- ***High-fiber foods (bran, some whole grains)***: Can slow absorption of medications such as thyroid hormone and iron supplements. Spread these foods out from medication times.
- ***Grapefruit and grapefruit juice***: Increases the potency (and sometimes toxicity) of many cholesterol and blood pressure medications. Avoid completely if you take drugs warned for this risk.
- ***Alcohol***: Widens side effects of muscle relaxants, pain relievers, and antidepressants. Even small amounts can worsen drowsiness or stomach trouble.
- ***Caffeinated beverages***: May increase jitteriness or GI upset with pain medications; also a mild diuretic, which may not be ideal with muscle weakness or cramping.

- ***Salt substitutes containing potassium***: If you're on diuretics or medications for high blood pressure, extra potassium can pose a risk.
- ***Tyramine-rich foods (aged cheeses, cured meats, fermented foods)***: A special alert only if taking older antidepressants (MAOIs); otherwise generally safe.
- ***Foods high in vitamin C (citrus, strawberries, tomatoes)***: Boosts iron absorption, making them beneficial when paired thoughtfully, but only at appropriate times.

Keep these "alert foods" posted on your fridge or meal-planning board as a quick check for new recipes, packaged foods, or when changing your medication schedule.

Drug-Food Interaction Symptom Log for Recognizing Adverse Events Tied to Meals

Spotting a medication-food interaction early can prevent bigger issues later. Many symptoms are subtle at first but become more obvious with careful tracking. Use a daily symptom log to record what you eat, when you take each medication, and how you feel afterward. Review this log weekly with your care team or whenever you notice changes in your energy, digestion, or mood.

Sample symptoms to watch for (and note the timing in relation to food/medication):

- ***Stomach pain, heartburn, or nausea shortly after taking medication***: May indicate you should take that medication with food, or need to change the type of meal you pair it with.
- ***Diarrhea, constipation, or unusual bowel changes***: Could signal a drug-food mismatch or the need to adjust fluid/fiber intake.
- ***Unusual fatigue, dizziness, new muscle weakness, or headaches***: May result from medications reaching too high or low a concentration because of meal timing or specific foods.
- ***Rash, swelling, or breathing issues***: Could signal a rare but serious food or medication allergy—seek immediate care.
- ***Poor symptom relief***: For example, ongoing pain or sleep issues despite medication may indicate absorption problems connected to your diet.
- ***Sudden changes in blood pressure or heart rate***: Especially concerning if using blood pressure medications, and certain foods or supplements have changed.
- ***Black, tarry stools or vomiting blood***: Potential sign of GI irritation or bleeding worth urgent evaluation, especially with NSAIDs or steroids.

For each log entry, record medication name, food or drink consumed, time taken, and your symptoms or impressions within 1-2 hours. Even subtle patterns (such as stomach cramping only when medication is taken on an empty stomach) are valuable for your healthcare provider.

Medication Administration Checklist With Built-In Meal/Snack Reminders

Building medication into your food routine is perhaps the most reliable way to prevent missed doses, confusion, or accidental doubling up. Use this simple checklist—a printable version can be displayed in your kitchen, bathroom, or wherever medications are stored:

Daily Medication Administration Checklist

For each scheduled dose, answer:

- *What medication am I taking?*
- *Does it need food, or must it be taken on an empty stomach?*
- *Which meal or snack will I pair it with today?*
- *Have I checked for any "alert foods" that could affect this dose?*

Before taking your medication:

- Double-check the time and confirm you have the right dose.
- Prepare your companion food or drink (if needed) and set aside water.

After taking your medication:

- Note the time and what you ate or drank.
- Log any unusual symptoms within the next two hours.

At the end of the day:

- Review your symptom log.
- Prepare medications, food pairings, and reminders for the next day.

Tips for Success:

- Use color-coded pillboxes (morning/with food, evening/empty stomach) for visual cues.
- Set alarms on your phone or use a physical timer for meal and medication pairings.
- Involve caregivers or family in double-checking doses and food matchups on days of high fatigue.
- Place a mini whiteboard or sticky note with daily "alert foods" or special instructions near your prep area for last-minute reminders.

Bringing It All Together

For people with PPS, making food the foundation of medication management isn't about making meals more complicated—it's about making life simpler, safer, and less stressful. A thoughtful approach to nutrient-drug interactions involves the entire care team: patient, caregivers, nutritionist, and pharmacist working together. Let food pave the way for more effective medications, and let well-timed medications support your best energy and symptom control. Balancing these elements may require experimentation, patient adjustments, and open dialogue, but the results can mean greater independence, fewer side effects, and a newfound sense of confidence in your daily self-care.

Sleep Optimization Framework for Post-Polio Fatigue (Frameworks)

For individuals with post-polio syndrome (PPS), restorative sleep is not a luxury—it is fundamental for reducing fatigue and maintaining day-to-day function. Unfortunately, PPS frequently disrupts sleep through muscular discomfort, breathing changes, increased nighttime awakenings, and the side effects of both medications and dietary habits. Yet, by consciously shaping what and when you eat and drink, along with optimizing your sleep environment, you can make meaningful improvements in sleep quality. This chapter presents a practical, step-by-step sleep optimization framework, tailored for the energy constraints and unique vulnerabilities of living with post-polio fatigue.

Pre-Bed Routine Template for Food and Fluid Timing

The timing of meals and beverages in the hours leading up to bedtime can make the difference between restful sleep and a disturbed night. For those with PPS, special care around pre-bed routines is warranted due to compromised muscle strength, slower digestive processes, and heightened sensitivity to even minor sleep disruptions.

To shape an effective pre-bed routine, consider these guidelines:

1. Aim to finish your last main meal at least three hours before bedtime. This gives your body adequate time to manage digestion and helps avoid reflux, nocturnal fullness, or discomfort that can increase awakenings.

2. Hydration is important throughout the day, but it's wise to taper off fluid intake about 90 minutes before lying down. This reduces the risk of nighttime bathroom trips—a well-known source of sleep fragmentation for people with limited mobility or muscle weakness.

3. Plan a small, optional snack approximately 30–60 minutes before going to bed if you struggle with nighttime hunger or blood sugar drops. This snack should be light, well-balanced, and composed of sleep-promoting nutrients (see the Late-Night Snack Menu below).

4. Avoid large meals, excessive sugar, or heavy/fatty foods in the two hours preceding sleep, as these can slow digestion further and provoke discomfort or indigestion, which is more pronounced for those with PPS.

5. Build relaxing, low-effort rituals—gentle stretching, slow breathing, or listening to calming music—into your routine so your body connects the act of winding down with the idea of sleep.

This routine minimizes late-night energy spikes, disruptive thirst, and nocturnal discomfort, creating conditions that support deeper, less interrupted rest.

Caffeine and Stimulant Intake Boundary Matrix

Caffeine and other stimulants are commonly used to fight fatigue, but they pose specific challenges for people living with PPS. While a morning cup of coffee or tea can offer a welcomed lift, stimulants linger longer in those with slowed metabolisms—intensifying sleep onset problems, nighttime awakenings, or restlessness.

Careful boundary-setting is especially critical for individuals who experience significant fatigue, mobility-related sleep disruption, or muscle cramps at night. Here's a simple decision matrix:

- ***Time-of-Day Boundaries***: Avoid caffeine and stimulant-containing foods and beverages (including coffee, black and green tea, cola, energy drinks, and chocolate) after 12:00 p.m. This allows your system enough time—often 8–12 hours—to clear these compounds before sleep, given the slower metabolism common among PPS survivors.

- ***Stimulant Dosage***: If you must have caffeine, limit yourself to one moderate cup (about 8 ounces) earlier in the day, as even modest afternoon intake can distill into significant sleep disturbance.
- ***Medication Synergy***: Some PPS-related medications—especially those used for fatigue or muscle cramps—may intensify the stimulating effects of caffeine or make its sleep-disrupting side effects worse. Check with your care team when adjusting your intake.
- ***"Hidden Stimulant" Awareness***: Watch for less obvious sources of caffeine and stimulants, such as decaf coffee (which can contain residual caffeine), certain pain relievers, and chocolate-based supplements or desserts. Read packaging and ask about these items whenever trying new foods or drinks.

By respecting these intake boundaries and keeping track of your caffeine exposure, you dramatically reduce the likelihood of stimulants magnifying both fatigue and insomnia—two of the most stubborn challenges for those with PPS.

Late-Night Snack Menu: Promoting Sleep Without Energy Spikes

Not all snacks are created equal when it comes to supporting sleep. For PPS survivors, the aim is to stave off hunger without flooding the system with fast-acting sugars or excessive calories, both of which can destabilize blood sugar or prompt nighttime wakefulness.

Here are sample late-night snack options that promote sleep while nourishing your body:

- ***Half a banana with a small spoon of peanut butter***: Bananas supply magnesium and potassium, which may ease muscle discomfort, while peanut butter adds protein and healthy fat for a gentle, steady energy release.
- ***Low-fat yogurt with a sprinkle of oats***: Yogurt contains tryptophan (an amino acid linked to sleep induction) and calcium, supporting muscle relaxation. A touch of oats supplies slow-digesting carbohydrates that help maintain stable overnight energy.
- ***A few whole-wheat crackers with reduced-fat cheese***: This pairing of complex carbs and modest protein keeps blood sugar balanced until morning.
- ***Warm milk (dairy or fortified plant-based)***: The warmth is soothing; the protein and calcium support sleep architecture.

- ***Sliced apple with almond butter***: Apple's fiber and almond's healthy fats keep hunger at bay without spiking energy late at night.

Snacks like these are designed to be easy to assemble and eat, gentle on compromised digestion, and unlikely to provoke a sugar rush or discomfort. Avoid sweets, chips, sugary cereals, and large portions. For those with swallowing or chewing issues, opt for smooth-textured yogurt, applesauce, or a blended smoothie using the same nutrient principles.

Bedroom Environment Adjustment Checklist

A supportive sleep environment is vital for everyone, but essential for people with PPS, who are often hypersensitive to changes in noise, light, temperature, or the physical layout of the bedroom. Small environmental missteps can lead to multiple awakenings and magnified fatigue the following day.

Use this checklist to create a more sleep-friendly setting:

- ☐ ***Noise Control***: Use white noise machines, earplugs, or soft music to mask external sounds that can trigger arousals—many with PPS become more noise-sensitive as their sleep becomes more fragmented.

- ☐ ***Light Management***: Install blackout curtains or use a sleep mask to block out ambient light, which can disrupt melatonin production and hinder sleep. Keep nightlights minimal or opt for dimmable bulbs to reduce sleep disruption if you require nighttime bathroom trips.
- ☐ ***Temperature Regulation***: Maintain a cool, comfortable temperature (usually between 60–67°F), as PPS can reduce the body's ability to regulate temperature and increase sensitivity to extremes.
- ☐ ***Bed Accessibility***: Ensure the bed is easy to approach and enter/exit. Arrange the room so pathways are clear, mobility aids are within reach, and there's a firm surface nearby for support during transfers. Consider installing bed rails or using assistive devices recommended by your occupational therapist.
- ☐ ***Mattress and Pillow Comfort***: Select a mattress and pillow that support your posture and relieve pressure—critical for those with muscle weakness or joint pain. Use wedge cushions or specialty pillows to reduce strain if you shift positions during the night.
- ☐ ***Organizing Essentials***: Place water bottles, medication, flashlight, and emergency contacts within arm's reach of the bed. This minimizes the need to move unnecessarily during the night.

Adjust as needed in collaboration with your care team to address changing mobility or comfort needs. Periodically review whether clutter, changing device positions, or deteriorating equipment is affecting your quality of sleep or ease of access.

Sleep Disturbance Trigger Journal Linked to Daily Nutrition Patterns

Understanding the relationship between what you eat, when you eat it, and your nightly sleep quality can unlock new levels of symptom management. Keeping a structured sleep disturbance trigger journal allows you to identify—and ultimately avoid—specific nutritional patterns that sabotage rest or amplify fatigue.

Set up your journal with daily entries like these:

- ***Bedtime and wake-up time***: To uncover shifts in sleep timing and their links to fatigue.
- ***Description and timing of evening meals/snacks***: Note what you ate and when, plus portion sizes.
- ***Fluid intake details***: Record all drinks after 5:00 p.m., specifying caffeine content, volume, and type.
- ***Quality and duration of sleep***: Rate how many times you woke up, how long it took to fall asleep, and how rested you felt on waking.

- ***Notable sleep interruptions***: Include details on needing the bathroom, muscle cramps, hunger, indigestion, or other disturbances.
- ***PPS symptom changes***: Record next-morning fatigue, muscle pain, or mood.

By reviewing several weeks of entries, you can spot links—such as increased awakenings after high-sodium or late, heavy meals, or restless sleep after afternoon chocolate or caffeine. Share this journal with your care team to refine both your nutrition and sleep strategies.

This system helps you pinpoint which evening eating routines calm your system versus those that interfere with vital rest. For many with PPS, consistently tracking and then adapting food and fluid patterns based on journal insights becomes a powerful tool to reduce nightly disruptions and manage fatigue systematically.

Bringing Your Framework Together

For people with post-polio syndrome, sleep is influenced by more than just a bedtime—nutrition, stimulant timing, bedroom setup, and symptom tracking are all deeply entwined. By integrating these targeted strategies, you can achieve:

1. Fewer nighttime awakenings due to discomfort, frequent urination, hunger, or environmental triggers.

2. More consistent sleep patterns by aligning caffeine, fluid, and food timings with your unique needs.
3. Proactive adaptation through journaling and adjustment, reducing day-to-day unpredictability in your energy and symptom levels.

Remember, PPS presents with individual variations; customizing this sleep optimization framework in collaboration with your clinical team will yield the best long-term results. As you apply these tools, your investment in better sleep pays over time—fewer fatigue flares, steadier moods, more reclaimed independence.

Adapting Your Plan for Flare-Ups and Bad Days (Troubleshooting)

Managing post-polio syndrome (PPS) means learning to adapt—sometimes on short notice. Even with strong daily routines, there will be times when fatigue surges, old symptoms worsen, or unexpected obstacles make your standard self-care plan feel out of reach. It's during these flare-ups and "bad days" that a proactive, easily-implemented troubleshooting strategy makes all the difference. This chapter equips you with ready-to-use tools and decision frameworks so you can maintain your nutrition and safety, even when your energy is at its lowest.

"Fatigue Flare" Nutrition Plan: Ultra-Simple, No-Effort Meal Options

When the effects of PPS intensify—whether because of illness, overexertion, or for no apparent reason—meal preparation can become overwhelmingly difficult. Muscle weakness, exhaustion, and pain all make standing or manipulating kitchen equipment a challenge. It's vital to have an ultra-simple nutrition plan specifically designed for these periods. The main goal during flares is to avoid energy crashes and sustain your body with basic nourishment, rather than striving for perfection or complex meal assembly.

Start by stocking your kitchen with shelf-stable and refrigerated options that require no cooking or extensive handling. Examples of "no-effort" meals and snacks for flare days include:

1. Ready-to-eat protein shakes or nutritional supplements. These are especially useful if chewing or swallowing is difficult or your appetite is diminished. Choose shakes that include iron, vitamin B12, and folic acid—nutrients frequently lacking in PPS diets and vital for energy levels and nerve health.

2. Pre-portioned, pre-cooked deli meats, cheese slices, or hummus paired with whole grain crackers or soft bread. These items are easy to assemble and require minimal physical effort.

3. Single-serve containers of unsweetened applesauce, yogurt, or cottage cheese. Opt for those fortified with vitamin D and calcium if possible, as these micronutrients support bone and neuromuscular health.

4. Canned tuna, salmon, or beans (no-salt added), which can be eaten directly from the can or simply paired with pre-washed leafy greens or microwavable pouch grains.

5. Cut fruit, pre-chopped vegetables, or baby carrots, along with small servings of nut butters or seed butters for added protein and healthy fats.

For even less effort, organize these no-cook items together in a designated drawer or basket within easy reach. Place clear labels so caregivers or family members can assist quickly.

Additional tips:

1. Hydration is especially important on fatigue flare days; keep bottles of water or electrolyte-rich drinks nearby to prevent dehydration, which can worsen PPS symptoms.
2. If swallowing becomes more difficult (a risk during PPS flare-ups), focus on smooth-textured foods and consider consulting your care team about thickeners or texture modifications.

Energy Conservation Task Prioritization Table for Daily ADLs (Activities of Daily Living) During Setbacks

With PPS, conserving your precious energy is crucial. On flare days, routine tasks like bathing, dressing, or preparing meals can quickly drain reserves, which may lead to increased weakness or risk of injury. Using a simple task prioritization table can help you identify which activities are truly essential and which can be postponed or delegated until you recover.

The following is an example of how to triage and delegate ADLs during a bad day:

- ***Absolute Essentials (must be performed)***: taking scheduled medications, consuming basic nourishment (even if simplified as above), hydration, and using the bathroom safely.
- ***Important but Deferrable***: full showers (opt for sponge baths as needed), changing clothes (unless soiled), nonurgent housework, administrative tasks.
- ***Low Priority/Defer or Delegate***: recreation and hobbies, extensive meal preparation, deep cleaning, errands, and any non-critical home maintenance.

In practice, check off the essentials first. For tasks in categories two and three, either delay or, if possible, rely on family, friends, or caregivers. On high-fatigue days, communicate early with your support team so expectations are clear and assistance is more easily secured.

If possible, prepare a printed table outlining your personal priorities for ADLs. Place it in a visible spot as a reminder for yourself and others involved in your care.

Pre-Scheduled Grocery Delivery and Takeout Menu for Contingency Nourishment

Nutrition matters most when it's hardest to maintain. Planning ahead for food access during setbacks can prevent skipped meals and nutritional deficiencies that quickly erode your strength. Pre-scheduling grocery deliveries and curating a reliable takeout menu are pragmatic ways to ensure you have nourishing options when fatigue interrupts your routine.

Strategies include:

1. Registering with an online grocery delivery service. Pre-select staple items (listed in your "fatigue flare" foods inventory) for quick re-ordering. Schedule regular (weekly or biweekly) deliveries, even if you often skip them, so you always have the option to avoid store trips when mobility or fatigue worsen.

2. Creating a printed or digital "emergency grocery list." Share this with a trusted neighbor, friend, or caregiver who can place orders or pick up supplies at short notice.

3. Curating a list of local takeout restaurants that offer healthy, soft, or easy-to-chew meals. Highlight menu choices that align with your energy support goals—such as broiled fish, vegetable-based soups, whole grain sides, and fruit cups. Avoid overly salty,

fatty, or sugary options, as these can worsen fatigue and disrupt digestion.

4. Keeping menus for these restaurants handy by the phone or in your kitchen. If possible, set up an online account with your preferred restaurant for one-click ordering.

Having these food access "backups" means you're less likely to skip meals or compromise nutrition when energy is scarce.

Rapid Symptom Escalation Action Checklist for Urgent Changes (Falls, Dysphagia, etc.)

During a post-polio flare, symptom escalation can occur rapidly—presenting serious risks, especially with falls, severe weakness, or sudden difficulty swallowing (dysphagia). Recognizing warning signs and acting quickly is critical for safety.

Prepare a Rapid Action Checklist that includes:

Signs meriting urgent action:

- ☐ Sudden, unexplained increase in weakness or inability to stand/walk.
- ☐ Loss of balance leading to a fall (with or without injury).
- ☐ Marked change in swallowing ability: coughing, choking, or sensation of food "sticking."

- ☐ Failure to pass urine or severe constipation with pain.
- ☐ New or intense pain, especially if different from normal PPS discomfort.
- ☐ Change in consciousness, slurred speech, or confusion.

Immediate Steps:

- ☐ Call for help—use medical alert systems, phone, or voice assistants.
- ☐ If you've fallen, do not try to get up alone; wait for help to reduce risk of further harm.
- ☐ For sudden swallowing problems, stop eating and drinking immediately to avoid choking; seek medical guidance.
- ☐ Record the exact time symptoms changed and what you experienced, as this will help health providers.
- ☐ If breathing becomes difficult, call emergency services immediately.

Keep this checklist accessible—in a purse, on the fridge, and share with your primary caregiver or family. Rapid response can prevent complications and ensure you receive timely care.

Signals When to Revert to Standard Plan: PPS-Specific Criteria List

Knowing when you are ready to transition out of your flare protocol and resume your usual routine helps restore confidence and reduces the risk of recurrent fatigue setbacks. A gradual, criteria-based approach is best.

Look for these PPS-specific signals before resuming your standard plan:

1. ***Return to baseline strength***: You can perform your usual ADLs (meals, personal care, basic movement) without marked increase in fatigue.

2. ***Consistent sleep***: You're able to sustain restorative sleep patterns for at least two consecutive nights.

3. ***Stable swallowing and digestion***: Meals go down smoothly, there's no increased coughing, or change in stool or urination patterns.

4. ***Appetite normalizes***: Interest in a wider range of foods returns, and you can safely manage more varied textures.

5. ***Absence of new or rapidly worsening symptoms***: No lingering confusion, balance problems, heightened pain, or other changes requiring medical review.

6. ***Emotional rebound***: Mood and motivation show improvement as your symptoms stabilize.

If you meet most or all of these criteria, begin, step by step, integrating your usual meal plans, activity pacing, and food prep routines. Continue to monitor energy patterns, and if uncertain, check in with your PPS care team before increasing activity or reverting entirely.

Integrating Flare Protocols into Daily Life

Many people with PPS find that clearly documented, visible plans for "bad days" reduce panic and support better self-management when symptoms worsen. Building your kitchen around ultra-simple meal options, automating grocery orders, having go-to restaurant menus, and prepping emergency routines make flare management less overwhelming for both you and your caregivers.

You may find it helpful to:

- Post your "fatigue flare" menu and ADL prioritization table on the fridge.
- Program phone reminders for regular hydration and nutrition, even on low-energy days.
- Keep the Rapid Symptom Escalation Checklist where it can be found at a moment's notice.
- Periodically rehearse flare plans with caregivers or family, so everyone is comfortable with roles and next steps.

Remember—flare plans are not a sign of setback, but of proactive, expert management. They empower you to continue nourishing your body and maintaining dignity and independence, even during the hardest days of PPS.

Caregiver and Family Coordination Toolkit (Tools)

Living well with post-polio syndrome (PPS) often requires a team approach. Fatigue, muscle weakness, and the unpredictability of symptoms mean that daily tasks—especially those related to food and self-care—can rarely rest on one person's shoulders for long. But as much as support is essential, clear communication and practical systems are what make support truly sustainable. This chapter gathers five easily adaptable tools to foster cooperation, reduce misunderstandings, and maximize everyone's energy in the PPS care environment. Use these as templates to share responsibility intentionally, protecting both your health and your relationships.

Shared Meal Prep and Shopping Calendar for Collaborative Delegation

For most people managing PPS, food decisions can never be entirely solitary. Whether you cook, shop, or rely on others for meals, keeping appointments, dietary needs, and shopping lists synchronized is critical to preventing both nutritional gaps and waste. That's where a shared meal prep and shopping calendar comes in.

A collaborative calendar supports everyone involved—as the person with PPS, as a primary caregiver, or as a family member who lends a hand now and then. Using a paper planner or a digital calendar, you track a week (or month) of meals, shopping needs, and division of labor. Here's how to get started:

1. List regular meal times and note who is responsible for each: breakfast may be solo, but dinner is shared, or perhaps weekends involve a different routine.

2. Record specific meal plans, noting which need advance prep (such as soaking beans, thawing meat, or chopping vegetables).

3. Assign shopping days and designate who will go, what stores they'll visit, and how groceries will be transported and stocked.

4. Identify who will prepare which meals and who will clean up.

5. Leave a column for "notes," where participants can flag shortages, leftovers, or remind each other of dietary changes.

This approach encourages everyone to share responsibility without assuming or guessing what the other person can do, want to do, or need help with. It helps prevent caregiver burnout by making delegation visible and normal. The collaborative element is especially vital in situations when PPS symptoms worsen and additional support is temporarily needed, such as during a flare-up, hospitalization, or emergency. Inviting everyone's participation also keeps the person with PPS involved in the planning and decision-making, reinforcing independence and agency as far as energy allows.

"My PPS Food Needs" One-Page Summary for Quick Caregiver Onboarding

Any time a new caregiver starts helping—whether a family member steps in for a week, a friend delivers meals, or a home health aide is assigned—the onboarding process can be stressful. Repeating or explaining specific dietary needs, food preparation preferences, restrictions, and routines can drain precious energy and open the door to unmet needs or mistakes.

That's why creating a "My PPS Food Needs" one-page summary is so powerful. This single sheet distills the essentials for anyone new to your care, making quick handovers and emergencies far less daunting. When crafting your summary, include the following sections:

- ***Brief diagnosis***: "I have post-polio syndrome. Fatigue, muscle weakness, and swallowing issues affect my eating."
- ***Key dietary requirements***: Outline necessary macronutrients, low-calorie adaptations, and specific protein or vegetable intake, as recommended for PPS management.
- ***Texture and prep needs***: Specify if foods must be easy to chew/swallow, portioned into small bites, or pureed; include any adaptive utensils or plate guards you use.
- ***Critical restrictions***: List allergies and foods to avoid (e.g., due to sodium, sugar, or fat content).
- ***Sample daily meal plan***: Show what a good food day looks like for you.
- Preferred cooking methods and dislikes.
- Reminders about hydration and meal spacing, given PPS-specific vulnerabilities to fatigue and dehydration.
- Emergency contacts for nutrition or medical concerns.

Updating and printing several copies of this summary lets you offer it to any friend, home care helper, or inpatient staff. It accelerates comfort, increases confidence, and reduces the odds of miscommunication. This document also reinforces to caregivers the non-negotiable aspects of your care, so your core dietary needs are never left to chance, even in unfamiliar circumstances.

Food Preferences and Dietary Restrictions Decision Sheet for Clear Communication

Individual preferences matter just as much as restrictions, especially with a diagnosis that can make every bite feel like a negotiation between pleasure, health, and convenience. A Food Preferences and Dietary Restrictions Decision Sheet puts everyone on the same page about what you like, what you tolerate, and what's off limits.

Start by splitting the sheet into "Preferences" and "Restrictions" columns:

- ***Preferences***: List favorite fruits, proteins, grains, and textures. Note cooking styles you enjoy (e.g., baked versus fried), go-to condiments, and comfort foods.
- ***Restrictions***: Itemize medical or wellness-related avoidances—such as low sodium, low added sugar, or low saturated/trans fats—highlighting reasons for each (e.g., blood pressure, digestive tolerance, or PPS-specific sensitivities).

For even more clarity, add a third column for "Sometimes Foods"—items you can have in moderation or with certain modifications (e.g., "plain yogurt, if low in sugar," or "white bread only when teeth are sore"). Stress the importance of checking serving sizes, portioning, and frequency, referencing any adaptations you make in line with PPS nutrition guidance.

Review this sheet with new and recurring caregivers and update it as preferences or doctor-advised restrictions change. This helps avoid the frustration that comes from unintentional risks or repeated meals that don't match your tastes. It also encourages everyone to use food labels and compare choices, fostering a culture of shared responsibility for healthy eating.

Weekly Food and Fatigue Status Report Template for Caregivers or Family Tracking

One of the underappreciated challenges in PPS care is the subtle, day-to-day shift in fatigue levels and how they interact with nutrition. A Weekly Food and Fatigue Status Report bridges this gap by documenting the interplay between meals, symptom severity, and functional ability.

This template can be used by the primary person with PPS, a family member, or a paid caregiver. Its primary sections include:

1. ***Daily fatigue score***: A number (e.g., 0–10) or descriptors for overall energy and alertness each day, cross-referenced to meals or snacks.
2. ***Main meals and snacks***: Record what was eaten, attention to portion sizes, and any changes in appetite.
3. ***Noted symptom changes***: Space for additional symptoms, e.g., muscle cramps, swallowing issues, or pain, which may relate to nutritional status.

4. ***Hydration***: Amount of fluid intake—important due to variable fluid needs in PPS.

5. ***Activity level***: List activities or exercise, if any, to see how exertion impacts both food intake and fatigue.

6. ***Observations***: Notes on the ease of eating/food prep and satisfaction with meals.

By structuring this report on a weekly basis, patterns become clearer (such as which foods promote better days, or whether fatigue spikes coincide with certain meals or missed snacks). Structured fatigue and well-being assessment is a recognized part of PPS management, with standard tools measuring symptom severity, quality of life, and physical function over time; incorporating such models into everyday status tracking makes care more responsive.

This log is especially useful for team discussions. When reviewing care at home, in clinic visits, or during transitions between care settings, this practical record provides concrete evidence to guide meal planning, troubleshooting, and even medication adjustments, building a truly individualized care plan.

Caregiver Self-Care Reminders Checklist for Sustainable Support

No system—no matter how finely crafted—will succeed if those providing care are running on empty themselves.

Sustainable PPS support requires that caregivers prioritize their own health and well-being just as vigilantly as the person they're helping. A Self-Care Reminders Checklist transforms this ideal into tangible action.

Here's a sample checklist for caregivers to use weekly or daily:

- ☐ Take regular breaks: Schedule small moments to rest, stretch, or step outside between caregiving and household tasks.
- ☐ Share or delegate responsibilities: Use the collaborative calendar so tasks don't pile on one person; ask for help when needed.
- ☐ Monitor your own stress: Check in with yourself using a stress or mood scale; if feeling overwhelmed, seek support or talk to someone you trust.
- ☐ Maintain your own nutrition and hydration: Prepare balanced meals for yourself and keep a water bottle accessible—healthy caregivers are more effective caregivers.
- ☐ Sleep hygiene: Prioritize regular, unbroken sleep whenever possible, and communicate if fatigue risks safe care provision.
- ☐ Know emergency protocols: Ensure you're clear on what to do if the person with PPS experiences sudden worsening of symptoms.

- ☐ Update knowledge: Review the "My PPS Food Needs" summary and Food Preferences sheet regularly so routines remain fresh and effective.
- ☐ Set aside personal time: Engage in an activity you enjoy, even for a few minutes each day, to recharge emotionally and physically.

Integrating these self-care reminders into the caregiving routine helps prevent burnout, resentment, and errors. It encourages a partnership approach, where the needs of both the person with PPS and their supporters are cared for with equal respect. Open conversations about limitations and about the need for substitute help during illness or absences are essential for resilience over the long haul.

Putting the Toolkit into Practice

These five tools are designed for immediate, flexible use—whether you're building your PPS support team from scratch or refining routines after years of experience. Adapting them to your context not only maintains nutritional quality and symptom stability but also preserves dignity and strengthens relationships.

In practical terms, begin by introducing one tool at a time. Start with the shared calendar and see how it improves meal planning transparency, then introduce the one-page summary for new helpers. As roles evolve, update the preferences sheet, use the fatigue and food status log for pattern tracking, and embed regular caregiver “check-in” moments using the self-care checklist.

By building a collaborative, documented, and caring environment centered on food and energy management, you transform daily living with PPS—from feeling isolated and overwhelmed toward empowered, sustainable teamwork. When everyone has a voice, and every routine is transparent, both nutrition and relationships flourish, laying the groundwork for a higher quality of life for years to come.

Conclusion: Turning a Food-First Plan Into Sustainable Everyday Action

Sustainable change in managing post-polio syndrome (PPS) fatigue is not about drastic overhauls or rigid diets. Instead, it's rooted in a series of small, intentional habit shifts that become part of everyday life. For those living with PPS, evidence shows that gradual changes—such as swapping out high-sugar snacks for fruit or slowly increasing your intake of fiber-rich foods—lead to far more lasting results than sudden, unsustainable efforts. Many individuals have found that breaking down goals into mini-steps—modifying one recipe, journaling daily intake, or adding a glass of water before each meal—builds confidence and reduces the risk of fatigue or discouragement that can come with attempting major life changes all at once.

This measured approach is particularly crucial given how fatigue often dominates the PPS experience. Research and lived experience alike highlight that when fatigue or muscle weakness is significant, even basic changes can feel overwhelming. For this reason, the most effective plans for PPS avoid pushing beyond personal energy limits, instead emphasizing "pacing"—the practice of making and sticking to minor, positive adjustments while recognizing early signs of fatigue or setbacks. For example: if regularly preparing meals becomes burdensome, the solution isn't necessarily to cook less nutritious meals, but rather to adapt recipes, batch cook on higher energy days, utilize leftovers creatively, or make smart use of prepared or no-cook foods. Exercise recommendations also follow this philosophy. Rather than aiming for an ambitious regimen, gentle stretching, light activity as tolerated, and regular check-ins with a physical therapist help maintain benefits without worsening fatigue or causing harm.

As your routines, symptoms, or living situations change—perhaps due to new care needs, outside help, or shifting abilities—it's important to adapt your food plan, rather than abandoning it. Regular self-reflection is key. Consider questions like: Are my current meal patterns helping or hindering my energy? Have appetite, swallowing, or mobility issues changed? Am I cooking more or relying on others for meals? Is there a new medication or therapy that affects my nutrient needs? With these changes, revisit and iterate your plan by making one or two targeted adjustments—such as incorporating more pre-cut produce, seeking lower-sodium options, or increasing hydration—then reassess after a week or two.

To help keep small changes on track and ensure your plan remains supportive, use this simple ongoing checklist:

- ☐ Keep a food journal or use your fatigue tracker to record meals, snacks, and corresponding energy levels.
- ☐ Compare similar foods when shopping to choose lower-fat, lower-sugar, or lower-sodium options as appropriate for you.
- ☐ Monitor for "red flag" fatigue signals—such as increased exhaustion, trouble swallowing, or worsening weakness—and pause or consult your care team if these arise.
- ☐ Stay hydrated by making water your main beverage and tracking intake, especially on low-energy days.
- ☐ Schedule regular reviews (e.g., every 4-6 weeks) with your support team or healthcare provider to re-evaluate and fine-tune your plan based on your current needs.

Managing PPS fatigue with a food-first approach is a dynamic, ongoing process. By choosing gradual adjustments, staying aware of your own signals, and working closely with your care team, you can adapt to the changing landscape of PPS and turn healthy intentions into daily action that lasts.

References and Helpful Links

Maynard, F. (2013). M. & Headley, J. L.. Post-Polio Syndrome: Pathophysiology and Management.

Maynard, F. (2013). M. & Headley, J. L.. Post-Polio Syndrome: Pathophysiology and Management.

Howard, R. (2005). S.. Post-polio syndrome: Pathogenesis and clinical aspects.

Smith, D. (2018). C.. Nutritional management of post-polio syndrome.

Mayo Clinic. (2022). Hyponatremia - Symptoms and Causes. Retrieved February 2, 2026, from https://www.mayoclinic.org/diseases-conditions/hyponatremia/symptoms-causes/syc-20373711

Centers for Disease Control and Prevention. (2020). Home and Recreational Safety: Falls Prevention. Retrieved February 2, 2026, from https://www.cdc.gov/falls/about/index.html

www.ingramcontent.com/pod-product-compliance
Lightning Source LLC
LaVergne TN
LVHW022005200926
848481LV00007B/2236
9798348521370